Keto for Beginners:

Essentials to Get Started with the Ketogenic Diet and Reset Your Metabolism in 14 Days

James Delgiovine

Table of Contents

publisher or the original author of this work can be in any fashion deemed liable for any hardship or damages that may befall them after undertaking information described herein.

Additionally, the information in the following pages is intended only for informational purposes and should thus be thought of as universal. As befitting its nature, it is presented without assurance regarding its continued validity or interim quality. Trademarks that are mentioned are done without written consent and can in no way be considered an endorsement from the trademark holder.

Introduction

Congratulations on downloading Keto for Beginners: Essentials to Get Started with the Ketogenic Diet and Reset Your Metabolism in 14 Days and thank you for doing so.

The following chapters will discuss the fundamentals of the Ketogenic Diet and will serve as a guide. Covering a wide range of topics that are perfect for the introductory reader, such as a sample shopping list, a list of foods to avoid, keys to understanding your body's metabolism, easy recipes, and a 14-day meal plan to help readers lose weight and reset their metabolism. Included are 21 secrets and facts about the keto diet and the process of ketosis. Also included is information on nutrition, and why making a commitment to the keto diet is synonymous with making a valuable commitment to your overall health.

There are plenty of books on this subject on the market, thanks again for choosing this one! Every effort was made to ensure it is full of as much useful information as possible; please enjoy!

Chapter 1: Fats Are NOT the Devil! Understanding Metabolism and Fundamentals of the Keto Diet

Imagine a car. The most beautiful car you can imagine: sleek, shiny, and it drives smooth. Imagine a house. Imagine your dream house. Maybe it overlooks a lake, maybe it's a cabin in the woods, or a luxe New York City penthouse. Now, imagine your body. What do all of these have in common? Fuel. If you keep loading up your car with low-quality fuel and wonder why it's not running smoothly even though you've checked everything else about the car, chances are that you're not loading up on the right fuel. Same goes for your house—you can design it as beautifully as you want, but if your electricity, plumbing, and heating aren't working properly, chances are you won't be able to fully enjoy all the beauty and benefits of your dream home. No, you don't need to repaint the walls or rearrange the furniture. Chances are, you need to go straight to the fuel source to experience and achieve the full changes that you want. The same logic goes for your body. Even if you're working out and getting enough exercise, even if you take good care of yourself on the outside, but still feel like you're holding on to excess weight or aren't able to experience the energy levels that you desire, the muscles that you want to build, or that overall feel-good mood, you need to examine what your body is using as fuel. If you don't change the fuel source, how can you expect to have different results? Yes, it's true: One of the key components to weight loss, maintaining a healthy weight, and to experiencing overall health is understanding how the body uses energy as fuel. So, what's fuel? I get it, you might ask. For cars, it's gasoline, electricity, or batteries. I know how that kind of energy works. For a home, it's a heating and electricity system, sourced from electricity plants, generators, solar power, or wind energy. Where does my body get its power? Where does my body find its energy? Food. There's a classic saying that goes: You are what you eat. Now, I don't mean that literally. But there is some truth to it! If you load up on healthy fats and essential vitamins and hydrate regularly with water, chances are you'll experience that inner glow and feel it on the outside, too. Healthy fats? What are you talking about? Isn't eating too much fat actually *unhealthy*?

Well, I hate love to break it to you. Fats aren't necessarily bad for you. They're actually fundamental to your health! Here's a quick rundown on how fats became the devil:

Picture the 90s, heroin chic, low-fat everything. You walk down the grocery aisle and notice everything from that pack of low-fat Activia to that low-fat milk to that low-fat, zero-calorie soda. Chances are, if you're trying to lose weight, the zero-calorie-low-fat tagline grabs your attention. As long as it's "diet," you want it. Other food items like avocados, nuts, or meat might be avoided like the plague. Anything that has more calories than 50, and that is loaded with fats? No, thanks. If you want to lose weight, you don't want anything that's loaded in fats. Common sense, eh? Well, not quite. Jump forward a couple decades. Bring yourself to now. Since then, it's been evident that fats do not necessarily make people fat—in fact, essential fats that are found in foods, such as avocados and almonds, are absolutely necessary for maintaining a slim frame and healthy, vibrant skin and hair. Everything that you might have avoided back then is exactly what you'd choose now. We've since learned that zero-calorie, low-fat foods typically contain close to no nutritional content. By going no-fat and restricting calories, you are denying yourself of the necessary energy and fuel sources that keep your body (and mind) running smoothly. Not only that, but without those necessary fats and essential amino acids, the body craves more carbs. (Ever wonder why when you go on a diet, you always feel hungry?) While certain carbohydrates found in fruits and vegetables are healthy, an excess amount of carbs found in candy, pasta, and processed foods tend to cause more weight gain and can result in lethargy, risks of disease and health conditions, and even mood disorders in extreme amounts. Enter the Ketogenic Diet. While our earliest ancestors ate a diet according to what they were able to forage, hunt, and gather, it's up to us now to make healthy decisions in the modern world.

A Brief History of the Keto Diet:

Here's what the Keto Diet is NOT:

- It's not considered vegan or vegetarian,

- It's not about calorie restriction,

- And it's not low-fat.

Now, here's what the Keto Diet IS:

- It's all about eating for your health and choosing meals according to their nutritious qualities,

- It's high in essential fats,

- It's low in carbs,

- And it's an excellent choice for rapid weight loss and resetting your metabolism

Since the 1920s, the keto diet has been practiced and encouraged by physicians and diet nutritionists. What makes the keto diet different from other diets (such as the Atkins or the Paleo diet) is that the keto diet is predominately high-fat, yet low-carb. This means that your body is using energy stores of carbs and producing ketones in the liver to be used as energy.

When the body consumes foods that are mostly high in carbs, it produces insulin and glucose. Essentially, glucose is a molecule that the body can easily convert into energy, and insulin is produced in the bloodstream to process the glucose and disperse it throughout the body.

Typically, when glucose is used as a primary energy source, fats are stored in the body because they are not needed. When you're eating a diet that is higher in carbs, glucose is used as the body's primary fuel for energy. If you lower your carb intake, then the body enters a process that is known as ketosis.

What is Ketosis?

When food intake is low, the body enters **Ketosis,** a natural state to help us survive when food intake is low. In the process of ketosis, **ketones** are produced from the breakdown of fats in the liver. Mostly, the main goal of the keto diet, when maintained properly, is to bring your body to this metabolic state. Although the body enters ketosis when the food intake is low, this does not mean that during the keto diet, you'll be restricting food and calorie intake. It merely says that you'll eliminate excess sources of carbs, so your body will take energy from the fat storage deposits and burn it off quicker. When you add more healthy fats to your diet and eliminate extra carbs, ketones are burned as the primary source of energy.

When you "go keto," you're putting your body into a state of ketosis: a metabolic state that occurs when most of the body's energy comes from ketone bodies in the blood, rather than from the sugar (also known as glucose).

When you're on the keto diet, your body thinks that it's fasting. Why? Since you've eliminated all those foods that include sugar and are heavy in carbs (like donuts and pasta), the glucose and sugar that is stored in your body is rapidly eliminated. To compensate for the lack of glucose and sugar, your body starts burning fat for energy rather than carbohydrates. This causes most people to lose their excess body weight very quickly, despite the fact that they are continuing to consume foods that are high in essential fats and eating enough calories. The ketosis process will also help to control the release of insulin and other hormones, which have roles in the development of diabetes and other health conditions. After going keto, your body may experience an instantaneous adjustment. After all, you've just radically shifted your diet and adjusted your fuel source!

The Rundown on Metabolism:

So what's metabolism all about, and how is it related to the keto-diet?

To convert food into energy, the body uses a combination of biochemical processes known as **Metabolism**. These metabolic processes include eating and digesting food, breathing, the methods of delivering nutrients through your bloodstream, how energy is used in your muscles, as well as your nerves and cells, and last but not least, the elimination of waste from your body.

In the context of dieting, metabolism isn't merely a chemical process. It is also a term that is used to describe the rate at which our bodies burn calories. You may have heard phrases like "slow or fast metabolism." This refers to the rate that your body converts food into energy (also known as calories). Our **metabolic rate** is the rate at which we burn calories or burn energy. The body will then use that converted energy to perform its daily functions.

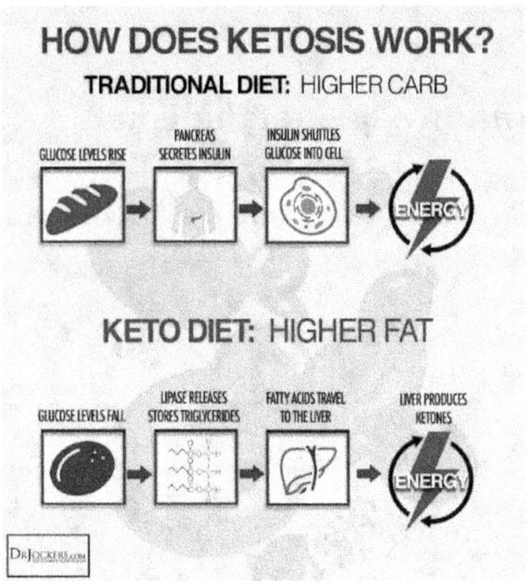

How to Achieve Ketosis:

Reaching ketosis is pretty simple, even though it may seem complicated due to the information we've explored earlier on in the chapter. So, to simplify the process, here's a list of ways your body can be induced into a ketogenic state.

- **Watch those carbs.** As we've explored in the earlier chapter, the keto diet is predominately low-carb. So make sure you're not consuming any of those sneaky grains like rice, pasta, bread, or cake!

- **Watch the amount of protein you're eating.** If you're used to the Atkins diet, chances are you're used to eating a lot of protein! However, having excess amounts of protein can lower ketosis levels. If you feel like your ketosis levels are too low, consider reducing the amount of protein you are consuming.

- **Don't worry about eating Fats!** You know it by now. The keto diet is a high-fat diet, so make sure you're eating enough fats. Even if you consider fasting (outlined below and in the next chapter), check in with yourself and make sure that you're not starving yourself. The keto diet is about nourishing your body with healthy foods, not about denial of essential nutrients.

- **Drink water.** Stay hydrated! Drinking enough water can reduce some of the side effects associated with starting the keto diet. If you're feeling hungry between meals, the chances are that you're also thirsty! So drink some water throughout the day, and you'll notice how beneficial hydration can be to your overall health.

- **Avoid snacking.** Too much snacking throughout the day is not conducive to weight loss, since you'll have fewer insulin spikes during the day. If you feel the urge to snack, consider having a glass of water or another beverage like some herbal tea or coffee. A handful of almonds or some raw veggies like carrots, cucumbers, or broccoli is also a healthy choice.

- **Consider Fasting.** As we will explore in the following chapter, fasting can be a quick method to elevate ketone levels throughout the day. There are different ways to fast, which include skipping meals, providing yourself with eating windows, or a full 24-hour cleanse. Here's a brief overview:

    - **Skip meals**. Consider skipping breakfast, lunch, or dinner if you want a quick fast.

    - **Give yourself an "Eating window."** An eating window is just what it sounds like. You give yourself a set time to eat (typically, a 4-to-7-hour window), and for the remaining hours, you fast. For example, your eating window could be something like from 10 a.m. to 3 p.m.

- **Twenty-four-hour cleanse**. For this extreme cleanse, you fast for an entire day. For the purposes of this book, this type of fast is not recommended.

- **Exercise!** Getting your body moving for at least 20-30 minutes a day can help aid weight loss while also boosting your mood. Going for a walk or a jog can work wonders and help balance blood sugar levels.

- **Supplement with Vitamins**. Consider supplementing fish oil, magnesium, potassium, or essential vitamins like vitamin D if you want an extra boost.

Chapter 2: 21 Secrets and Facts About the Keto Diet

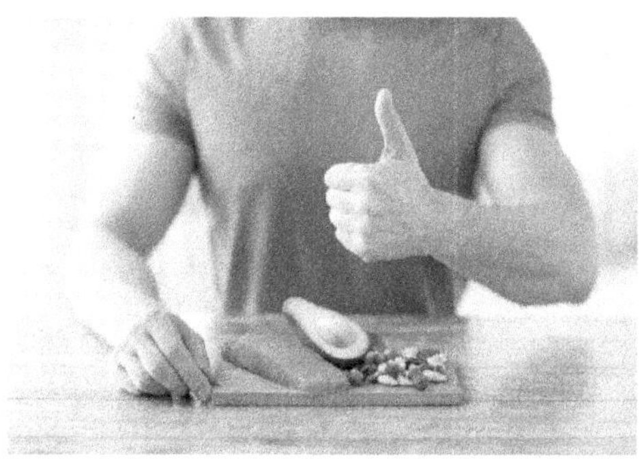

Q: Have you ever struggled with maintaining a healthy weight, with sculpting muscle, high blood sugar, vision problems, acne, digestive disorders such as IBS, acid stomach reflux, or heartburn? What about chronic migraines, depression, or lethargy? If you answered yes and had experienced any of the health conditions listed above, you might be wondering what these health conditions have in common... and how a simple change could solve a variety of ailments associated with the health conditions listed above. Based on what we've learned about in the previous chapters, I think you already know the answer!

(Drum roll please)

A: It's no surprise by now that the Keto Diet is a tried, tested and accurate solution to improving and reducing symptoms associated with migraines, low energy levels, digestive disorders, and any other symptoms related to the health conditions listed above. Ready to unlock the secret code, otherwise known as the Keto Diet? Read on.

21 Secrets and Facts About the Keto Diet:

1. Aids weight loss. On keto, your insulin levels drop, which makes it easier to lose weight.

2. Help sculpt muscle

3. Helps maintain vision (especially with patients who have glaucoma)

4. Lowers the Risk of Heart Disease

5. Reduces Risk of Type 2 Diabetes and Lowers Blood Sugar. By removing excess carbohydrates from one's diet, one can prevent excess insulin from being released. When insulin levels are in balance, blood sugars are normalized. Keto naturally lowers blood sugar levels

6. Provides Protection Against Cancer

7. Anti-Aging Benefits and Aids Longevity. The essential healthy fats found in a lot of foods like avocados and almonds help promote and protect skin elasticity and smoothness, vibrant hair, and strong nails.

8. Allows Reverse Neurological Disorders and Brain Disease

9. Helps Clear Skin. That shows a probable connection between high-carb eating and increased acne, so it's likely that keto can help.

10. Helps Reset Metabolism

11. Reduces Acid Stomach Reflux and Severity of Heartburn Symptoms

12. Increases Brain Function

13. For those who suffer from IBS, the Keto diet may relieve abdominal pain and cramping.

14. Improves Immunity

15. Lowers Inflammation

16. Stabilizes Energy Levels and Improves Performance.

17. Decreases migraines and intensity of headaches

18. Potential Mood Stabilizer

19. Helps Improve Side Effects Associated with Autism

20. Helps Manage Symptoms of those with Multiple Sclerosis (MS)

21. Fuel for the brain and helps with Mental Focus. Many people use the ketogenic diet *specifically* for the increased mental performance. An increased intake of fatty acids (such as omega 3, found in fish) helps your brain function.

Chapter 3: Advice for the Keto-Lifestyle

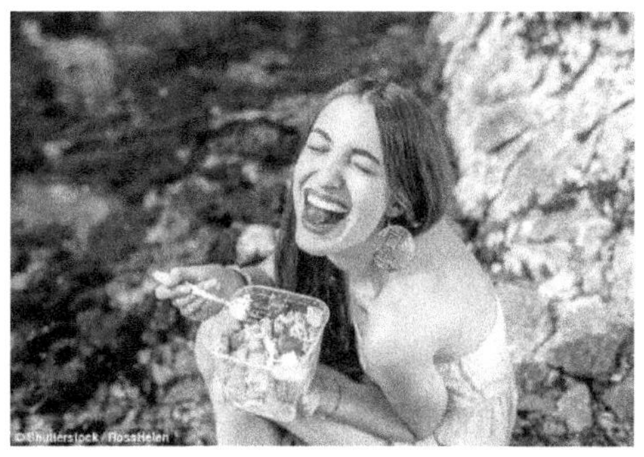

The Keto Diet is not only a diet but also a lifestyle. As you go about your daily life, you are surrounded by many choices to make, such as where to eat and what to eat. Fortunately, the keto diet is adaptable to many different situations. At most restaurants, there are often keto-friendly options on the menu.

Everyday dieting recommends between 20 and 30 g of net carbs. The more you reduce your carbohydrate intake and lower your glucose levels, the better the overall results will be regarding your health and weight loss goals. If your goal is weight loss, try to measure both your total carbs and net carbs. Remember to keep having protein (found in eggs and nondairy milk alternatives like almond milk, veggies, fish, and meat).

What's A Net Carb?

Net carbs = your total dietary carbohydrates – the entire fiber.

Where can you find the best net carbs? Dark leafy greens are the ideal choice for vegetables. Combine most of your meals with good sources of protein and veggies, with a side of fat. Here are some simple sample ideas: Chicken breast with a side of green beans and a squeeze of lemon, or consider topping a steak with some butter, and sauté some spinach in olive oil.

Here's a list of the most common low-carb vegetables.

Vegetable	Amount	Net Carbs
Raw Spinach	½ cup	0.1

Romaine Lettuce	½ cup	0.2
Steamed Cauliflower	½ cup	0.9
Raw Green Cabbage	½ cup	1.1
Raw Cauliflower	½ cup	1.4
Broccoli	½ cup	2
Collard Greens	½ cup	2
Steamed Kale	½ cup	2.1
Steamed Green Beans	½ cup	2.9

What is Intermittent Fasting?

Intermittent fasting creates a limit on your calorie intake since you're controlling the amount of food intake. Naturally, your body can only handle a certain amount of food at one time, so intermittent fasting is a handy method to help people who are trying to lose weight. Wait, I thought you said no calorie restriction! Well, intermittent fasting is not necessarily calorie restriction—it's about making sure you're eating the healthiest foods possible, with the highest nutritional content, at controlled intervals. As your body adjusts to fasting, you won't be as hungry as you used to be.

In this fasting state, your body breaks down extra fat and uses it for energy. When your body reaches ketosis, the levels of glucose leave your bloodstream at a rapid pace since the fats are being used as energy.

In intermittent fasting, your stored fat is used for energy. Be careful, though. Intense fasting can also lead to a yo-yo effect, causing you to put the pounds back on after you've finished fasting. To prevent this from happening, you need to eat some more fat according to your metabolism and engaging in a consistent exercise regime to avoid storing the excess fats.

Potential Risks

- Dramatically reducing your intake of carbs may cause you to feel hunger during the first 2-3 weeks of starting the diet. If this is the case, make sure you stay hydrated and have some healthy snacks (like a handful of almonds) throughout the day.

- You may experience what is commonly known as "the keto flu," which is headaches and fatigue due to the sudden loss of water weight. This sudden loss of water weight can cause dehydration, so be sure to stay hydrated! Consider taking some electrolytes in your water, too. These can be found in Emergen-C vitamin packets that dissolve in water or other similar brands.

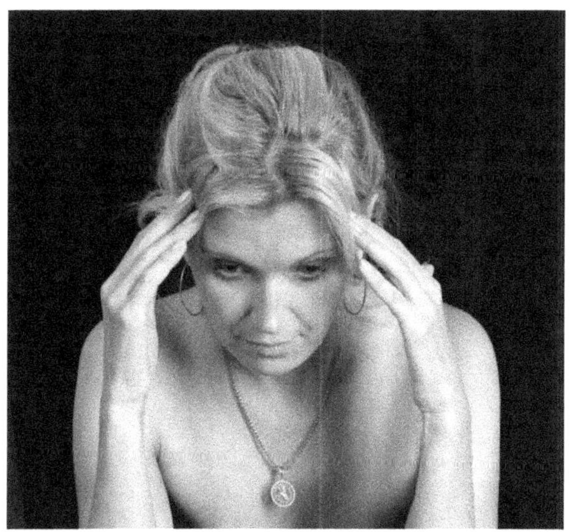

- Other risks are kidney stones, vitamin and mineral deficiencies, decreased bone mineral density, and gastrointestinal trouble. *To avoid these risks, be sure to consult a healthcare professional before beginning the diet. If you are deficient in essential vitamins and minerals, consider supplementing with vitamins while you're on a diet, to avoid further deficiencies.*

- While some fats can be healthy, be careful not to increase your intake of unhealthy trans and saturated fats. These fats are found in foods like red meat, poultry skin, butter, and cheese. Consuming these foods in very high amounts can lead to higher cholesterol rates and elevated risks of heart disease. That being said, be sure to balance out meals of cheese, red meat, butter, and poultry with other delicious options like vegetables, fish, and nuts.

Who Should Not Follow a Keto Diet

- If you have diabetes (Type 1 or Type 2), blood sugar conditions like hypoglycemia, have kidney disease, or any liver, pancreatic or kidney issues or situations.

- If you have type 1 diabetes and take medicine for diabetes.

- If you require medications for diabetes or any of the health conditions listed above, consult first with a doctor.

- If you have Muscular Dystrophy or other conditions, the keto-diet may severely distress the pancreas, liver or kidneys.

- If you are pregnant, trying to become pregnant, or are currently nursing.

- If you are underweight or have an eating disorder

- Children and Teens under 18 years old

- If you are in recovery or anticipating a surgery

- If you have a pre-existing medical condition and are unsure about how the diet may affect the prescriptions you are taking, consult with your doctor before beginning the diet.

- If you are feverish or physically ill.

- If you have a history of mental illness and mental health conditions, speak with your doctor first.

Chapter 4: Understanding the Components of Easy Recipes and Balanced Meals

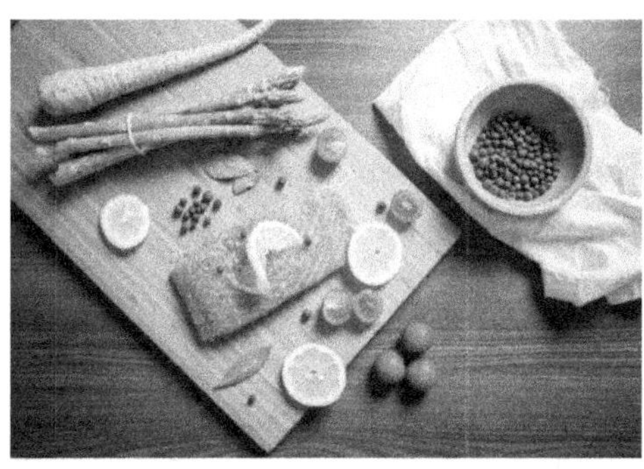

Ever wanted to jump-start your keto-diet, but didn't know where to get started? These following chapters will show you a multitude of possibilities and recipes that are all super delicious, affordable, and... you guessed it... ketogenic! Who said that diets had to be restrictive, and who said that cooking had to be hard? Let's debunk those dieting and cooking myths, by getting hands-on in the kitchen. One of the many benefits of a Keto-Diet include an abundance of vegetables, and proteins to choose from. See the sample shopping list below, and enjoy the rainbow of foods that are available to you:

Sample Shopping List:

Dairy and Eggs:

- Eggs

- Butter

- Sour Cream

- Whipped Cream

- Cheese (such as cheddar, parmesan, Swiss, etc.)

- And more

Meat and Fish:

- Bacon

- Ground Beef

- Salmon

- Trout

- Tuna

- Pork rinds

- Anchovies

- Fowl (such as chicken and turkey)

- Lamb

- And more

Vegetables and Fruits:

- Avocados
- Lemons
- Limes
- Tomatoes
- Spinach
- Cauliflower
- Broccoli
- Watercress
- Brussel Sprouts
- Bell Peppers
- Eggplant
- Cucumbers
- Kale
- Asparagus
- Cabbage
- Zucchini
- Green beans
- Olives

- Berries (strawberries, blueberries, blackberries, raspberries, etc.) in moderation

- Nuts (walnuts, pecans, almonds, brazil nuts, macadamia nuts, pine nuts, peanuts, etc.). Eat cashews and pistachios sparingly.

- Coconut

- And more

Note: Consume vegetables ground below ground more sparingly. These include:

- Parsnips

- Beet Root

- Onion

- Carrots

Spices, Herbs, Oils and Condiments:

- Basil

- Cilantro

- Parsley

- Rosemary

- Paprika

- Chives

- Dill

- Garlic

- Mint

- Cinnamon

- Thyme

- Cloves

- Black Pepper

- Cayenne pepper

- Oregano

- Turmeric

- Cumin

- Ginger

- Nutmeg

- Chia Seeds

- Cacao Powder

- Protein Powders

- MCT Oil

- Sunflower Oil

- Vegetable Oil

- Olive Oil

- Coconut Oil

- Olive Oil

- Ketchup

- Dijon Mustard

- Mayonnaise

- Peanut Butter

- Almond Butter (including other nut butters)

- Sesame Tahini

- Soy Sauce

- And more

Drinks:

- Red Wine (in moderation)

- Tea

- Coffee

- Water

Foods to Avoid:

- Beans

- Rice

- Pasta

- Sugar

- Milk

- Fruits

- Bread

- Soda

- Fruit juice

- Candy (chocolate bars, gummies, etc.)

- Beer

- Potatoes

- Processed foods

- Fast foods

Majority of the foods you eat will be fats (70%), followed by proteins (25%), and carbs (5%). Despite being a high-fat diet, the keto-diet is considered low-carb for this reason.

According to the keto diet, a balanced meal will include the essential elements illustrated in the following food chart:

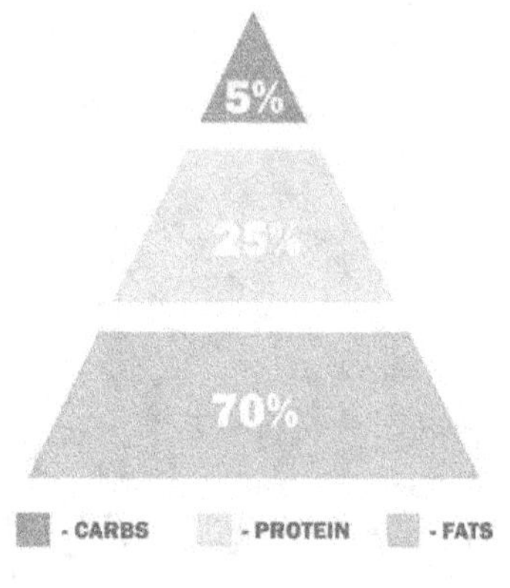

Now that we have a sample shopping list, and some examples of foods to avoid, how about some sample recipes?

Chapter 5: Jumpstarting Your Ketogenic Diet

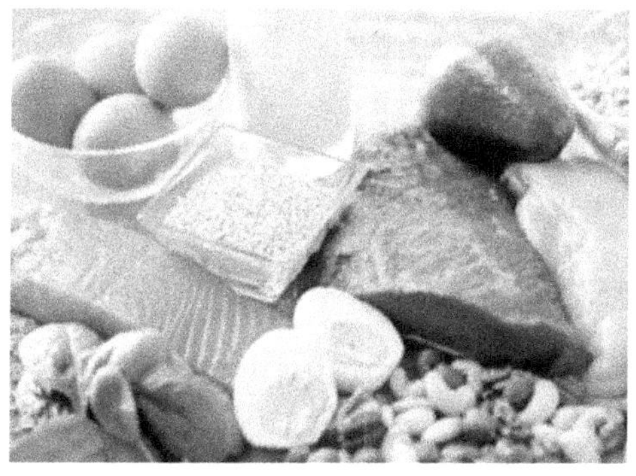

Now that we've explored the fundamentals of the keto-diet let's put all that we've learned into action! Here's a 14-day meal plan, to help you kick-start the keto diet and to reset your body's metabolism. Please note that if you are new to the diet, you may experience certain side effects as your body detoxes and adjusts. These side effects may include frequent urination, dizziness, drowsiness, sugar cravings, low blood sugar, digestive issues like constipation or diarrhea as the body detoxes, changes in sleep, flu-like symptoms, headaches and/or confusion. These symptoms, although they are unpleasant, are often signs that the body is detoxing as the body burns through the excess glucose in the muscles and the liver and releasing excess water. Hang in there... These side effects should only last for a few days at most. If these side effects continue for more than a few days, however, please consult a doctor or licensed healthcare professional. Many of these recipe ideas have been adapted from helpful websites such as Diet Doctor and Dr. Axe. Many thanks to the online platforms and generous contributors who have provided culinary inspiration and made the inclusion of these recipes accessible and possible.

Additional tips for beginning the 14 Day Meal Plan:

- When doing the meal plan, feel free to mix and match recipes according to your taste. For example, if you enjoy a special breakfast, you may repeat it as much as you like. What matters is that you're enjoying the process and getting your health back on track in the process.

- Simplify your meals: Cook two servings for lunch or dinner today and refrigerate the second serving for your meal tomorrow.

- If you're not hungry at breakfast, consider skipping the meal and having a hearty lunch instead. In moderation, intermittent fasting not only saves you time and money, but also it raises your ketone levels.

A Note on the Meals:

The recipes provided are easy and at the beginner level. Some recipes such as the Pad Thai, Cauliflower Grilled Cheese Sandwiches, Smoked Salmon Cloud Biscuits, Salmon and Egg Brekkies and the Quiche have been added in for readers who may want a little challenge. If you prefer less cooking, feel free to repeat some of the non-cooking options, such as the salads, and meat and cheese plates. As you get cooking in the kitchen, I'm confident you'll discover the many benefits and rewards of cooking the keto-way!

14- Day Meal Plan

Day 1:

Breakfast

Steak and Eggs

This recipe makes 1 serving, requires about 10 minutes of preparation, and 5 minutes of cooking time.

The serving size is 1 portion; it contains:

44 g Protein

3 g Carbs

36 g Fats

What's in It

- Butter (1 tbsp)
- Eggs (3)
- Avocado (1 sliced)
- Sirloin (4 oz, sliced)
- Salt (to taste)
- Pepper (to taste)

How it's Made

- In a pan, melt the butter and fry the eggs sunny-side up. Season with salt and pepper.

- In a separate pan, cook the sirloin as desired.

- Place the eggs and sirloin onto a plate. Slice the pieces of sirloin.

- Add in the sliced pieces of avocado. Serve and enjoy!

Lunch

BLT Salad

This recipe makes 2 servings and requires about 15 minutes of preparation.

The serving size is 1 salad; it contains:

17.5 g Protein

18 g Carbs

18 g Fats

7 g Fiber

What's in It

- Kale (3 cups, shredded and without stems)

- Bacon (4 strips, chopped)

- Avocado (2 oz, sliced)

- Grape Tomatoes (10, halved)

- Extra Virgin Olive Oil (2 tsp)

- Vinegar (1 tsp)

- Salt (¼ tsp)

- Pepper (to taste)

How it's Made

- Mix the salt, olive oil, kale, and vinegar with the kale in a bowl, until the kale has been coated and softened.

- Halve the grape tomatoes, and slice the avocado

- Cook the bacon

- Boil the eggs in a pot so that they are soft or hard-boiled, depending on taste.

- Set aside two bowls and divide the kale and the eggs accordingly. Add the tomatoes, the bacon, salt, pepper, and the avocado. Serve and enjoy!

Dinner

Frittatas

This recipe makes 4 servings, requires about 15 minutes of preparation, and requires about 35 minutes of cooking time.

The serving size is 1 frittata; it contains:

22 g Protein

7 g Carbs

20 g Fats

What's in It

- Eggs (10 large)

- Bacon (5 slices, cut into small chunks)

- Baby Spinach Leaves (4 oz)

- Small Tomatoes (2 sliced thin)

- Red Onion (1 large)

- Mustard (3 tsp)

- Salt (to taste)

- Pepper (to taste)

- Basil leaves (to taste)

- Butter (1 tbsp)

How it's Made

- Preheat the oven to 350 degrees Fahrenheit.

- In a bowl, make the egg and mustard mixture. Whisk the mustard, eggs, salt, and pepper.

- Heat the butter on an ovenproof skillet over medium heat. Add the bacon and the onion, and cook for about 5 to six minutes, until the onion is golden brown.

- Add the spinach leaves and cook until wilted.

- Add the egg and mustard mixture into the skillet and cook until it begins to harden.

- Place the tomatoes on top.

- Cook until the frittata sets around the edges, but make sure the center is runny in the middle.

- Place the skillet in the oven for another 30 minutes.

- Take the frittata out from the oven, decorate with basil leaves. Serve and enjoy!

Day 2:

Breakfast

Eggs, Avocado, and Ground Beef Bowl

This recipe makes 1 serving and requires about 15-20 minutes of preparation.

The serving size is 1 salad; it contains:

8.5 g Fiber

25.9 g Carbs

37.9 g Fats

What's in It

- Onion (1 small, diced)
- Eggs (2, lightly beaten)
- Avocado (1, diced)
- Mushrooms (7 medium, sliced)
- Black Olives (11, sliced)
- Ground Beef (1 portion, according to taste)
- Smoked Paprika (½ tbs)
- Coconut Oil (alternative: olive oil, according to taste)
- Salt (to taste)
- Pepper (to taste)

- Parsley (leaves, to taste)

How it's Made

- Heat a drizzle of oil in a skillet over medium heat. Add the mushrooms and onions. Sprinkle with salt and pepper. Cook for about 2 or 3 minutes, until the vegetables have softened.

- Add the paprika and the ground beef. Cook for about 10 minutes.

- Once the beef is no longer pink, remove the beef onto a plate.

- Now add the eggs into the skillet and scramble them.

- Once the eggs are scrambled to your liking, put the beef back into the skillet.

- Add the avocado and the olives. Cook for just under a minute.

- Set aside a bowl and transfer the food from the skillet. Add salt, pepper, and parsley leaves if desired. Serve, and enjoy!

Lunch

Chicken Soup -- Ideal for leftovers

This recipe makes 4 servings and requires about 30 minutes of cooking time.

The serving size is 1 bowl of soup; it contains:

33 g Protein

4 g Carbs

40 g Fats

What's in It

- Butter (2 oz)

- Mushrooms (3 oz, sliced)

- Celery (1 stalk)

- Carrot (½ medium sized)

- Dried Onion (1 tbsp, minced)

- Garlic (1 clove, minced)

- Chicken Broth (4 cups)

- Parsley (1 tsp, minced)

- Salt (to taste)

- Pepper (to taste)

- Rotisserie Chicken (¾ cooked, shredded)

- Green Cabbage (1 cup, sliced)

How it's Made

- In a large pot, melt the butter.

- Cut the celery and the mushrooms into small pieces.

- Add the celery, mushrooms, onion, and garlic into the pot. Cook for about 3-5 minutes.

- Pour in the broth. Add the carrot. Sprinkle with salt and pepper to taste. Simmer.

- When the vegetables are tender, add the chicken and cabbage.

- Simmer for about 10 minutes, until the chicken and cabbage are tender.

- Set aside a bowl and transfer the soup from the pot. Serve, and enjoy!

Dinner

Pork Chops

This recipe makes 1 serving and requires about 30 minutes of preparation and cooking.

The serving size is 1 plate; it contains:

54 g Protein

6 g Carbs

73 g Fats

What's in It

- Pork Chop (1)

- Green Beans (4 oz)

- Butter (½ oz)

- Salt (to taste)

- Pepper (to taste)

- Parsley (optional)

- Lemon (optional, a squeeze)

How it's Made

- Prepare the pork chops by cutting small slits in the sides so that the chops will stay flat while frying. Sprinkle the chops with some pepper and salt.

- Place the pork chops and the butter into a frying pan. Cook on medium-high heat and fry the chops on both sides for about 5 minutes.

- Once the chops have fried, remove them from the pan and transfer to another plate.

- In the same frying pan, cook the green beans on medium-high heat for a few minutes. Add some salt and pepper to the green beans as you cook.

- You'll know the green beans are ready when they are soft yet still crunchy to bite.

- Transfer the green beans onto the same plate as the pork chops. Sprinkle with salt, pepper, and a squeeze of lemon as desired.

- Serve, and enjoy!

Day 3:

Breakfast

Mushroom Omelet

This recipe makes 1 serving and requires about 5-10 minutes of preparation.

The serving size is 1 omelet; it contains:

25 g Protein

4 g Carbs

43 g Fats

What's in It

- Eggs (3)

- Butter (1 oz)

- Onion (⅕)

- Mushrooms (3)

- Cheese (shredded, 1 oz)

- Salt (to taste)

- Pepper (to taste)

How it's Made

- In a large bowl, crack the eggs and whisk with a fork. Add salt and pepper to taste.

- In a frying pan, melt the butter. Pour in the egg mixture.

- As the eggs cook, add the cheese, mushroom, and onion.

- Once the omelet has cooked, place it on a plate. Serve and enjoy!

Lunch

Grilled Cheese Cauliflower Sandwiches

By day three, you're probably missing that nice taste of freshly toasted bread. Don't worry, for here's an alternative to bread that has a lot of nutritional benefits! The main ingredient? Cauliflower!

This recipe makes 2 servings and requires about 40-45 minutes of preparation and cooking time.

The serving size is 1 sandwich. Each slice of cauliflower bread contains:

7.4 g Carbs

4g Fats

What's in It

- Egg (1)

- Cauliflower (1 head, stem removed. Chopped in small florets)

- Cheddar Cheese (2 slices)

- Parmesan Cheese (½ cup, shredded)

- Italian herb seasoning (1 tsp)

- Salt (to taste)

How it's Made

- Preheat oven to 450F. Remove stem from cauliflower, cut into small pieces. Place it into food processor and pulse until the cauliflower pieces resemble crumbs.

- Take the cauliflower out of the food processor, and place into a safe microwave bowl. Microwave for 2 minutes until the cauliflower is soft and hot.

- Take the cauliflower out of the microwave, and mix. Then put it back into the microwave for another 3 minutes. Take the cauliflower out of the microwave and mix again so that the cauliflower is evenly cooked. Cook in the microwave for 5 minutes. By now, the cauliflower should be becoming drier. Finally, microwave for yet another 5 minutes until the cauliflower is a little moist but dry enough to be crumpled up. Keep in mind that the cauliflower will be used as the bread of the grilled cheese.

- Cool the cauliflower for a few minutes in the same bowl. Once it has cooled, mix in the egg and cheese, until the consistency becomes smooth. Add in seasoning.

- Form the dough into slices resembling cut loaves of bread. Line a large baking sheet with parchment paper and place the slices of cauliflower bread onto it.

- Bake cauliflower bread for about 15-20 minutes. When the cauliflower bread is golden brown, take it out of the oven and cool a few minutes.

- Slide the cauliflower bread off of parchment paper using a spatula. Time to assemble your grilled cheese sandwiches!

- Place the loaves of cauliflower bread and cook on the stove top, just like you would normally cook a grilled cheese. Another option is to place the grilled cheese sandwiches back into the oven and broil for several minutes (5-10) until the bread is toasted and the cheese has melted. Once ready, serve and enjoy!

Dinner

For dinner today, consider having some of the leftover chicken soup from yesterday.

Chicken Soup Leftovers

This recipe makes 1-2 servings and requires about 5-10 minutes of cooking time.

The serving size is 1 bowl of soup; it contains:

33 g Protein

4 g Carbs

40 g Fats

What's in It

- Butter (2 oz)

- Mushrooms (3 oz, sliced)

- Celery (1 stalk)

- Carrot (½ medium sized)

- Dried Onion (1 tbsp, minced)

- Garlic (1 clove, minced)

- Chicken Broth (4 cups)

- Parsley (1 tsp, minced)

- Salt (to taste)

- Pepper (to taste)

- Rotisserie Chicken (¾ cooked, shredded)

- Green Cabbage (1 cup, sliced)

How it's Made

- Place the chicken soup into a pot on the stove, on medium heat for several minutes, until hot. Or, place the soup into a microwave-safe bowl and microwave until hot.

- Serve, and enjoy!

Day 4:

Breakfast

Smoked Salmon and Eggs Brekkies

This recipe makes 2 servings and requires about 30 minutes of preparation and cooking time.

The serving size is 1 brekkie. Each brekkie contains:

0.96 g Carbs

23.53 g Fats

18.25 g Proteins

What's in It

- *Eggs (2)*

- *Smoked salmon (4 oz, sliced)*

- *Salted Butter (½ tbsp)*

- *Chives (2 tbsp, chopped)*

- *Salt (to taste)*

- *Pepper (to taste)*

For the Hollandaise Sauce:

- *Salted butter (2 tbsp)*

- *Egg Yolk (1, separated from the white)*

- *Dijon mustard (¼ tsp)*

- *Lemon (½ of juice)*

- *Water (½ tbsp, add more if the sauce is too thick)*

- *Salt (to taste)*

How it's Made

- Prepare all ingredients. Make sure ingredients are at room temperature.

- Boil a small pot of water on the stove. When the water has boiled, add in the two eggs and boil for 10-12 minutes, until completely hard-boiled.

- As the eggs boil, dice the salmon into small pieces.

- Heat 2 teaspoons of butter in a skillet over high heat. Once the butter has melted up, add half of the cut salmon pieces into the pan. Cook until the pieces are crisp. Once crisp, set aside.

- By now, the eggs should have boiled. Run the eggs in cold water so that they are cooled before you begin to peel them.

- Once cooled, peel the eggs and put them in a dish. Use a fork to mash the eggs.

- Now begin your hollandaise sauce.

- Place a pot with about a couple cups of water onto the stove. Let the water simmer.

- Melt the 2 tablespoons of butter in the microwave for 30-60 seconds. Make sure the butter is melted but not hot. Set aside to cool.

- In a large heat-safe bowl whisk the egg yolk, lemon juice, Dijon mustard and some salt together until you see air bubbles in the mixture.

- Put the bowl with egg mixture over the pot with the simmering water to create a double boiler. Make sure that the water does not touch the bottom of the bowl. Use medium heat and whisk the mixture until it thickens.

- Once the mixture starts thickening, pour in the melted butter while you stir with a whisk. Keep stirring as you pour to avoid clumps. Once all of the butter is added, place the bowl back onto the pot so that the mixture can thicken further.

- When the sauce is thick enough, remove the bowl from over the pot and set it aside. Add some water if you think that the sauce is too thick, but keep in mind that a thick consistency is desired.

- Let the hollandaise to cool until it reaches room temperature.

- Take the raw salmon, hollandaise, and the chives. Mix all these together with the mashed egg until a firm mixture is formed. You don't want this to be too wet so limit the hollandaise if you see this happening.

- Once the ingredients have been combined, separate the mixture into four pieces and roll into balls.

- Mix your remaining chives and the crispy salmon together and roll your brekkies in this to coat. Serve, and enjoy!

Lunch

Goat Cheese Salad

This recipe makes 1 serving and requires about 10 minutes of preparation.

The serving size is 1 plate of salad. Each plate contains:

73 g Fats

37 g Protein

3 g Carbs

What's in It

- *Baby Spinach (a handful or two)*

- *Goat Cheese (5 oz)*

- *Balsamic Vinegar (to taste)*

- *Butter (1 oz)*

- *Pumpkin Seeds (at least 2 tbsp, to taste)*

- *Salt (to taste)*

How it's Made

- Preheat the oven to 400 degrees Fahrenheit. Grease a baking dish and add in the goat cheese. Put into oven and bake for about 10 minutes.

- As the goat cheese bakes, toast the pumpkin seeds in a small pan for a couple of minutes, until fragrant. These seeds will be used to garnish the salad.

- Add in some butter and balsamic vinegar to the frying pan and mix in with the seeds on low heat for a few more minutes.

- Take the goat cheese out of the oven.

- Assemble the baby spinach onto a plate. Add the goat cheese and the balsamic butter pumpkin seeds.

- Serve, and enjoy!

Dinner

If you're a fan of burgers, don't worry: You don't have to give them up. Well, not quite... (just the bun). Open your mind and your taste buds, to this awesome alternative:

Icebergers

This recipe makes 4 servings and requires about 30 minutes of preparation

The serving size is 1 burger; it contains:

8 g Protein

134 mg Phosphorus

115 mg Sodium

162 mg Potassium

What's in It

- Iceberg Lettuce (1 large head)

- Bacon (4 slices)

- Red Onion (1, sliced)

- Tomato (1, sliced)

- Cheddar Cheese (2 oz.)

- Ground Beef (1 lb.)

- Salt (to taste)

- Pepper (to taste)

How it's Made

- To create the shape of the buns, slice the iceberg lettuce into large rounds from the edges of the lettuce.

- Place the slices of bacon into a large skillet and cook on medium heat until crispy.

- Line a plate with paper towels, and once the bacon is cooked, place the bacon on the plate to cool and drain. Be sure to leave the bacon fat in the pan.

- Add the onions to the pan and cook each side for about 3 minutes. Once the onions are cooked, set aside and wipe the skillet.

- Shape the ground beef into medium patties, place onto the skillet, and cook on medium-high heat. Season with salt and pepper.

- Add a slice of cheese to each patty. Cover the skillet with a lid until the cheese melts (should be about 1 minutes). Remove from heat.

- Now it's time to build the burgers! To construct each one, top one iceberg with the cooked cheeseburger, a slice of bacon, and a

tomato slice. Place on the second iceberg
round. Serve, and enjoy!

Day 5:

Breakfast

Bacon and Eggs

Ahh, now here's a simple classic! Who would've thought that your favorite childhood breakfast is also ketogenic?

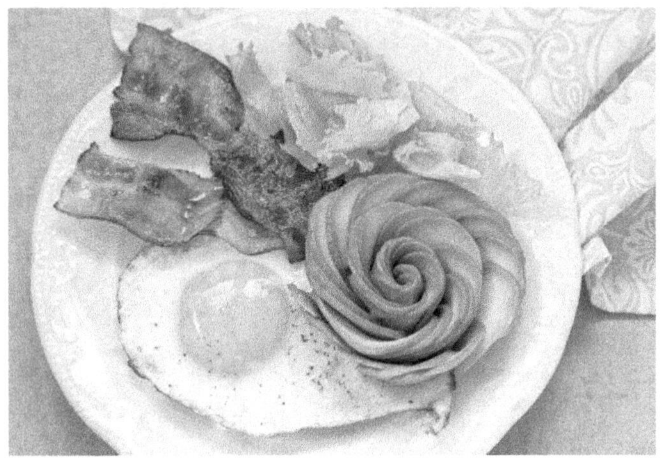

This recipe makes 1 serving and requires about 5-10 minutes of preparation and cooking time.

The serving size is 1 portion of eggs, bacon, avocado. Each portion contains:

22 g Fats

15 g Protein

1 g Carbs

What's in It

- *Eggs (2)*

- *Bacon (2-3 slices, 1 ½ oz)*

- *Cherry Tomatoes (optional)*

- *Avocado (1, sliced)*

- *Lettuce (optional)*

- *Salt (to taste)*

- *Pepper (to taste)*

How it's Made

- Fry the bacon in a skillet over medium heat until the bacon is crisp.

- Once crisp, remove from skillet and place on a separate plate.

- Cook the eggs as you like them best -- sunny side up, scrambled, or omelet.

- Once the eggs are cooked, place onto a plate with the bacon and sliced avocado. If you'd like, add some lettuce and cherry tomatoes for taste, and a pinch of salt and pepper. Serve, and enjoy!

Lunch

Roast Beef and Cheddar Plate

 This recipe makes 1 serving and requires about 5 minutes of preparation.

The serving size is 1 plate. Each plate contains:

98 g Fats

38 g Protein

6 g Carbs

What's in It

- *Roast Beef (3 oz, sliced, deli cut)*

- *Cheddar Cheese (2 oz)*

- *Mayonnaise (4 tbsp, or to taste)*

- *Mustard (½ tbsp, or to taste)*

- *Lettuce (1 oz)*

- *Radishes (3)*

- *Salt (to taste)*

- *Pepper (to taste)*

How it's Made

- Assemble the roast beef onto a plate. Add the slices of cheddar cheese, roughly chopped lettuce, and sliced radishes. Sprinkle with salt and pepper. Add some mayonnaise and mustard according to taste.

- Serve, and enjoy!

Dinner

Tex-Mex Burger

This recipe makes 1 serving and requires about 5-10 minutes of preparation.

The serving size is 1 plate. Each plate contains:

101 g Fats

50 g Protein

8 g Carbs

What's in It

- *Ground beef (5⅓ oz)*
- *Water (cold, 1 tbsp)*
- *Tex-Mex seasoning (½ tbsp)*
- *Pickled jalapeños (1 tbsp)*
- *Mayonnaise (4 T)*
- *Mexican cheese (2 oz, sliced)*
- *Avocado (1)*
- *Arugula lettuce (1 oz)*
- *Olive oil (1 tbsp, or according to taste)*
- *Salt (to taste)*
- *Pepper (to taste)*

How it's Made

- Mix the ground beef with Tex-Mex seasoning and water. Form into one burger patty.

- Brush the burger patty with olive oil, and grill (or fry) each side for about 3-4 minutes.

- When the burger was cooked according to your taste, put it on a plate and surround it with the sliced avocado, jalapeños, arugula, Mexican cheese, and mayonnaise. Pour on a small amount of olive oil for enhanced taste. Serve, and enjoy!

Day 6

Breakfast

Toast-less, Deconstructed Avocado Sandwich

Keep it simple this morning by slicing up a fresh, ripe avocado and drizzling some olive oil, lemon or lime juice across it. Sprinkle with salt and add some cherry tomatoes on the side if desired. All the benefits, just without the bread.

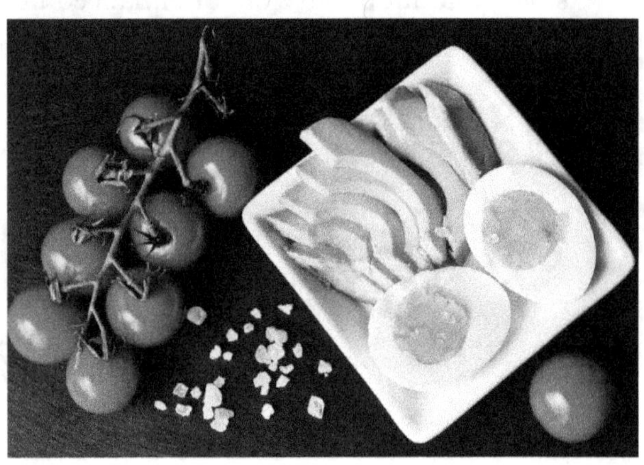

Lunch

Smoked Salmon Cloud Biscuits

This recipe makes 4 servings and requires about 5 minutes of preparation, and 15 minutes of cook time.

The serving size is 1 biscuit; it contains:

30 g Protein

6 g Carbs

41 g Fats

3 g Sugar

4g Fibre

What's in It

- Egg (1)

- Cheddar cheese (3/4 cup)

- Smoked salmon (8 oz)

- Red Onion (2 tbsp)

- Heavy Cream (1 tbsp)

- Almond Flour (4 oz)

- Baking Powder (1 tsp)

- Cayenne Pepper (1 tsp)

- Cream Cheese (4 oz)

- Arugula (rocket, a handful)

- Lemon (1, juiced)

- Dill (optional, if desired)

How it's Made

- Set oven to 350°F

- In a large bowl, add the almond flour and the cheddar cheese. Stir, while mixing in the baking powder and cayenne pepper

- In a separate bowl, crack and whisk the egg.

- In the bowl with the flour and cheese, mix in the whisked egg mixture.

- Once the egg has been mixed in, stir in the cream.

- On a baking sheet, scoop out the mixture, so it forms patties.

- Place the tray with the patties into the oven for 15 minutes.

- Take the patties out from the oven, and cool for a couple of minutes.

- Once cooled, cut the biscuits in half.

- Now it's time to construct the sandwich. Spread the cream cheese, rocket, and salmon. Add a little lemon juice and a lemon wedge for decoration. Serve and enjoy!

Dinner

Steak Stir-Fry

This recipe makes 1 serving and requires about 20 minutes total cooking and preparation time.

The serving size is 1 plate. Each plate contains:

75 g Fats

40 g Protein

10 g Carbs

What's in It

- *Ribeye Steaks (6 oz)*

- *Broccoli (4 oz)*

- *Onion (½, sliced)*

- *Butter (2 oz)*

- *Soy Sauce (to taste)*

- *Salt (to taste)*

- *Pepper (to taste)*

How it's Made

- Chop the onion and the broccoli. Slice the ribeye steak.

- In a wok (or a frying pan), heat up some butter on medium-high. Add the steak and cook until brown on both sides. Sprinkle with salt and pepper as you cook.

- Once the steak has been cooked to your liking, place it on another plate and set aside.

- In the same wok (or frying pan,) toss in the broccoli and the onion. If needed, add in some more butter.

- Once the onion and broccoli have cooked to your liking, add the steak back into the wok and mix. If you wish, add in some soy sauce and add some more butter.

- Once the veggies and steak have been mixed, transfer the stir-fry onto a separate plate or bowl. Serve, and enjoy!

Day 7

Breakfast

Devilled Eggs

This recipe makes 8 servings and requires about 10 minutes of preparation

What's in It

- Eggs (6 hard boiled)

- Avocado (1 large)

- Bacon (3 T, broken into bits)

- Garlic (1 t, minced)

- Shallot (1 t, diced)

- Lemon (1, juiced)

- Salt (to taste)

- Pepper (to taste)

How's it Made

- Boil the eggs and let them cool.

- Once the eggs have cooled, remove the shell and slice the eggs in half.

- Remove the yolks from the egg and place them into a large bowl.

- Mix in the garlic, shallot, lemon juice, bacon and avocado into the bowl, along with the egg yolks. Mash until the mixture becomes smooth.

- Using a small spoon, spoon the avocado and yolk mixture back into the egg.

- Serve and enjoy!

Lunch

Salami and Cheese Plate

This recipe makes 1 serving and requires about 5 minutes of preparation time.

The serving size is 1 plate. Each plate contains:

113 g Fats

38 g Protein

5 g Carbs

What's in It

- *Brie Cheese (3 oz)*

- *Lettuce (1 oz)*

- *Avocado (1, sliced)*

- *Cherry Tomatoes (optional)*

- *Salami (2 oz)*

- *Nuts (a handful, according to taste: almonds, macadamia, or walnuts).*

- *Salt (to taste)*

- *Pepper (to taste)*

- *Olive oil (2 tbsp)*

How it's Made

- Place the cheese on a plate. Roughly chop the lettuce and slice the avocado into wedges. Add the salami, nuts, cherry tomatoes, salt, and pepper. Drizzle on the olive oil according to taste.

- Serve, and enjoy!

Dinner

Bacon Burgers

This recipe makes 1 serving and requires about 5 minutes of preparation time.

The serving size is 1 burger. Each burger contains:

76 g Fats

42 g Protein

7 g Carbs

What's in It

- *Bacon (1¾ oz, or a couple slices)*

- *Ground beef (5⅓ oz)*

- *Water (½ tablespoon cold)*

- *Red Onion (1/2 , thinly sliced)*

- *Chilli paste (½ teaspoon)*

- *Salt (to taste)*

- *Pepper (to taste)*

- *Olive Oil (to brush onto the burgers)*

For serving

- *Dill pickles (¾ oz, to taste)*

- *Cheddar cheese (sliced, ¾ oz or to taste)*

- *Lettuce (¾ oz)*

- *Tomato (1 small, thinly sliced)*

- *Mayonnaise (to taste)*

- *Ketchup (to taste)*

How it's Made

- Separate a slice of bacon for the burger. Chop the other slice of bacon into small pieces.

- Add some cold water and mix the bacon bits with the ground beef and chili paste. Form into a burger patty shape with your hands.

- Wrap the reserved slice of bacon around the burger patty. Brush with olive oil. Place onto the grill (or fry) for 5-10 minutes, until the meat has cooked according to your preference.

- Once cooked, place the burger patty onto a plate. Add the pickles, sliced tomato, lettuce and onions onto the plate. Add some mayonnaise or ketchup, according to taste.

- Serve, and enjoy!

Day 8

Breakfast

Avocados and Salmon

This recipe makes 1 serving and requires about 5 minutes of preparation time.

The serving size is 1 portion of avocado and salmon. Each portion contains:

22 g Fats

15 g Protein

1 g Carbs

What's in It

- *Avocado (1, sliced in half)*

- *Smoked Salmon (3 oz)*

- *Mayonnaise (6 tbsp) -- (Alternative choice: sour cream)*

- *Cherry Tomatoes (optional)*

- *Lemon (½, a squeeze)*

- *Salt (to taste)*

- *Pepper (to taste)*

How it's Made

- Cut the avocado in half, remove the pit, and peel the outer coat. In the hollow of the center where the pit was, add some mayonnaise (or sour cream -- according to taste).

- Place the bits of smoked salmon onto the mayonnaise and avocado.

- Squeeze the lemon onto the avocado and salmon, and sprinkle with some salt and pepper according to taste.

- Serve, and enjoy!

Lunch

Deconstructed Greek Salad Plate

This recipe makes 1 serving and requires about 5 minutes of preparation time.

The serving size is 1 plate. Each plate contains:

102 g Fats

62 g Protein

9 g Carbs

What's in It

- *Chicken (½ lb., cooked)*
- *Black Olives (4-6)*
- *Olive Oil (to taste)*
- *Tomato (1, sliced in wedges)*
- *Iceberg lettuce (a handful, roughly chopped)*
- *Feta Cheese (3 oz)*
- *Lemon (½, a squeeze)*
- *Salt (to taste)*
- *Pepper (to taste)*

How it's Made

- Assemble the plate. Place the pieces of chicken on the plate, along with the tomatoes, cheese, iceberg lettuce, and black olives. Drizzle some olive oil on the plate and squeeze half a lemon if desired. Add a pinch of salt and pepper according to taste.

- Serve, and enjoy!

Dinner

Pad Thai

This recipe makes 4 servings and requires about 20 minutes of preparation, and 10 minutes of cook time.

The serving size is 1 bowl; it contains:

90 g Protein

13 g Carbs

34 g Fats

5 g Fibre

What's in It

- Eggs (3, beaten lightly)

- Chicken tenders (2 lbs)

- Chicken broth (⅓ cup)

- Zucchini (4, spiralled)

- Scallion (½ cup, chopped)

- Tamari (2 tbsp)

- Rice vinegar (1 tbsp)

- Peanut Butter (3 tbsp)

- Peanut Oil (2 tbsp)

- Garlic Powder (⅛ tsp)

- Garlic (2 cloves, minced)

- Ground Ginger (⅛ tsp)

- Red pepper flakes (to taste)

- Salt (to taste)

- Pepper (to taste)

- Bean Sprouts (½ cup)

- Peanuts (½ cup crushed, for decoration)

- Lime (1, cut into wedges)

How it's Made

- In a bowl, mix the ginger, garlic powder, salt, and black pepper. Place the chicken tenders into the bowl and mix until the tenders are coated.

- Heat the peanut oil over medium-high heat in a medium skillet. Add the chicken tenders and cook for about 3 minutes, until each side is reasonably cooked. Take the chicken out of the pan and cut the tenders into ¼-inch-thick slices. Set aside.

- Scramble the eggs in the pan for about 1 minute. Once they are scrambled to your liking, take the scrambled eggs out of the pan and set aside.

- Turn down the heat to medium-low and pour in the chicken broth. Add the peanut butter, vinegar, tamari, scallion, garlic. Sprinkle in red pepper flakes to taste. Mix together, cooking for about 3 minutes.

- Put the chicken slices, scrambled eggs, zucchini noodles and bean sprouts back into the skillet. Coat the chicken, eggs, and zucchini with the sauce. Cook for approximately 1 minute.

- Place the chicken pad Thai into a bowl and serve. Add the peanuts and lime wedges to taste. Serve, and enjoy!

Day 9

Breakfast

Steaming Cuppa Coffee

Looking to kickstart your morning the keto way? Consider brewing up a keto-style coffee!

This recipe makes 1 serving and requires about 5 minutes of preparation time.

The serving size is 1 cup; it contains:

1 g Protein

0 g Carbs

38 g Fats

What's in It

- Unsalted butter (2 tbsp)

- Coconut oil (1 tbsp) -- Alternative choice MCT Oil

- Coffee (1 cup, brewed).

How it's Made

- Mix the freshly brewed coffee, oil, and unsalted butter in a blender. Blend until the consistency is frothy and smooth.

- Serve, and enjoy!

Lunch

Ripped Green Salad

Love your greens with an extra punch? Then this recipe is just what you're looking for.

This recipe makes 1 serving and requires about 10 minutes of preparation.

The serving size is 1 salad.

What's in It

- *Bean Sprouts (a handful)*

- *Avocado (1, cut into wedges)*

- *Spinach Leaves (a handful)*

- *Arugula (rocket, a handful)*

- *Olive Oil (3 tbsp)*

- *Salt (to taste)*

- *Lemon (a squeeze)*

How it's Made

- In a bowl, mix the bean sprouts, avocado, spinach, and rocket with the olive oil and lemon. Sprinkle in salt as needed.

- Voila! You're ready to serve. Enjoy!

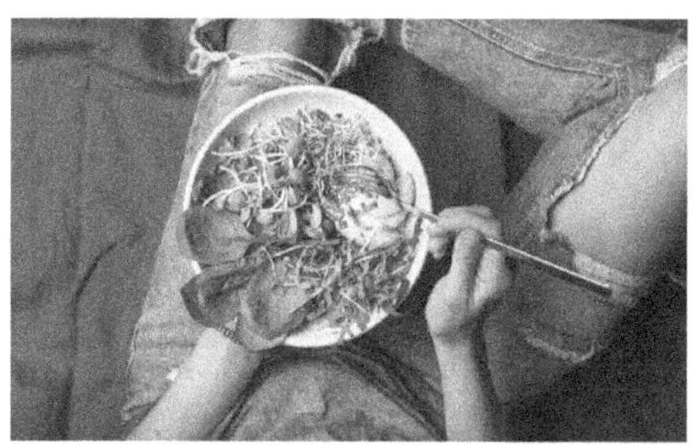

Dinner

For dinner, consider having some of the leftover Pad Thai from yesterday.

Pad Thai Leftovers

This recipe makes 4 servings and requires about 20 minutes of preparation, and 10 minutes of cook time.

The serving size is 1 bowl; it contains:

90 g Protein

13 g Carbs

34 g Fats

5 g Fibre

What's in It

- Eggs (3, beaten lightly)

- Chicken tenders (2 lbs)

- Chicken broth (⅓ cup)

- Zucchini (4, spiralled)

- Scallion (½ cup, chopped)

- Tamari (2 tbsp)

- Rice vinegar (1 tbsp)

- Peanut Butter (3 tbsp)

- Peanut Oil (2 tbsp)

- Garlic Powder (⅛ tsp)

- Garlic (2 cloves, minced)

- Ground Ginger (⅛ tsp)

- Red pepper flakes (to taste)

- Salt (to taste)

- Pepper (to taste)

- Bean Sprouts (½ cup)

- Peanuts (½ cup crushed, for decoration)

- Lime (1, cut into wedges)

How it's Made

- In a bowl, mix the ginger, garlic powder, salt, and black pepper. Place the chicken tenders into the bowl and mix until the tenders are coated.

- Heat the peanut oil over medium-high heat in a medium skillet. Add the chicken tenders and cook for about 3 minutes, until each side is reasonably cooked. Take the chicken out of the pan and cut the tenders into ¼-inch-thick slices. Set aside.

- Scramble the eggs in the pan for about 1 minute. Once they are scrambled to your liking, take the scrambled eggs out of the pan and set aside.

- Turn down the heat to medium-low and pour in the chicken broth. Add the peanut butter, vinegar, tamari, scallion, garlic. Sprinkle in red pepper flakes to taste. Mix together, cooking for about 3 minutes.

- Put the chicken slices, scrambled eggs, zucchini noodles and bean sprouts back into the skillet. Coat the chicken, eggs, and zucchini with the sauce. Cook for approximately 1 minute.

- Place the chicken pad Thai into a bowl and serve. Add the peanuts and lime wedges to taste. Serve, and enjoy!

Day 10

For Day 10, Breakfast and Lunch will be combined into a healthy and nutritious brunch. Kickstart your morning with a freshly brewed coffee or tea, and let's get started!

Quiche

This recipe makes 4 servings and requires about 40 minutes.

The serving size is 1 portion; it contains:

7 g Fiber

6 g Carbs

50 g Fats

What's in It

- *Coconut oil (1 tbsp) -- alternative butter*

- *Onion (1, chopped)*

- *Spinach (1 bag, chopped).*

- *Eggs (8, beaten)*

- *Raw Cheese (3 cups, shredded)*

- *Salt (to taste)*

- *Pepper (to taste)*

How it's Made

- Preheat oven to 350 degrees F. Grease a pie pan with coconut oil (or butter, according to taste).

- Put onions and coconut oil in a saucepan over medium heat and cook until the onions are soft. Next, mix in the spinach and cook until it wilts. By now, the excess moisture should be evaporated.

- In another bowl, crack and beat the eggs, and add the cheese. Sprinkle with salt and pepper. Add spinach mixture to the bowl and mix together.

- Transfer the mixture into the pie pan and bake for 30 minutes in the oven

- Once the quiche is baked, let cool for a couple of minutes. Then serve and enjoy!

Dinner

Sesame Chicken

This recipe makes 4 servings and requires about 30 minutes.

The serving size is 1 portion; it contains:

7 g Fiber

6 g Carbs

50 g Fats

What's in It

- *Chicken thigh (1 lb.)*

- *Sesame seeds (3 tbsp)*

- *Almond flour (4 oz)*

- *Red pepper flakes (optional)*

- *Eggs (2)*

- *Broccoli (7 oz)*

- *Salt (to taste)*

- *Pepper (to taste)*

- *Heavy cream (3 oz)*

- *Red bell peppers (2 oz, thinly sliced)*

- *Sesame oil (2 tbsp)*

- *Soy sauce (3 tbsp)*

- *Spring onion (3 oz, sliced)*

- *Lime (1, juiced)*

How it's Made

- Preheat oven to 400°F

- In a bowl add the sesame seeds, almond flour. Sprinkle salt, pepper, and chili flakes to taste.

- In another bowl, crack the eggs and add cream. Whisk the eggs and the cream together.

- Now it's time to prepare the chicken thighs. Dip the chicken thigh into the egg and cream mixture. Next, dip the chicken thigh into the sesame and almond flour mix.

- Repeat this process for all the chicken thighs.

- Place the prepared chicken thighs onto a tray and put into the oven for 30 minutes.

- Steam broccoli cooked. To prevent the broccoli from cooking further, you can put them in a bowl of cold water.

- Take the chicken thighs out from the oven. Drizzle sesame oil and soy sauce.

- Place chicken thighs and steamed vegetables onto a plate.

- Sprinkle sliced spring onions and red bell pepper onto the dish. Serve with lime and enjoy!

Day 11

Breakfast

Keto Cheese Rolls

These cheese rolls are the perfect snack to have alongside the breakfast options we have explored previously in this chapter. Consider whipping up a nice omelet, some eggs sunny-side up, or some bacon. These cheese rolls will add some extra taste!

This recipe makes 2 servings and requires about 5 minutes.

The serving size is 1 cheese roll; it contains:

13 g Protein

2 g Carbs

31 g Fats

What's in It

- *Butter (⅙ oz)*

- *Cheddar Cheese (4 oz, sliced. alternative choice: Provolone Cheese)*

- *Salt (to taste)*

- *Herbs (to taste, such as parsley or paprika)*

How it's Made

- Place the pieces of sliced cheese onto a clean surface area.

- Place the butter on a cutting board and cut into very thin slices.

- Place a small amount of butter on the cheese slices and roll up.

- Sprinkle with salt, desired herbs, and spices. Serve, and enjoy!

Lunch

Kale Salad

What's in It

- *Kale (9oz)*

- *Limes (2, juiced)*

- *Olive oil (2 tsp)*

- *Beetroots (2)*

- *Pine nuts (3 ½ oz)*

- *Salt (to taste)*

- *Pepper (to taste)*

How it's Made:

- Tear the kale leaves from their stalks and put into a salad bowl.

- Make a dressing out of lime juice and olive oil by mixing the two ingredients together and add this to the salad bowl.

- Using your hands, work the dressing into the kale leaves. After a couple of minutes, the kale should be thoroughly coated with the dressing.

- Now it's time to peel the beetroots. Once peeled, grate the beetroots using a greater.

- Heat up the pine nuts in a small frying pan for a few minutes, until they are fragrant and toasted. Add the pine nuts and the grated beetroot to the kale. Mix, and sprinkle with salt and pepper. Serve, and enjoy!

Dinner

For dinner today, consider having some of
the leftover sesame chicken from yesterday.
You can toss it into a salad or heat it up.

Day 12

For day 12, let's take a trip around the world. Begin the day with a fresh Italian breakfast plate. For lunch, prepare a nutritious beef and sesame Asian salad, and for dinner, take a trip to France to enjoy a classic bacon and ham omelet.

Breakfast

Mozzarella and Prosciutto Plate

This recipe makes 1 serving and requires about 5 minutes. Consider pairing with a sunny-side-up an egg if you want an extra protein boost!

The serving size is 1 plate; it contains:

40 g Protein

8 g Carbs

69 g Fats

What's in It

- *Tomato (1, sliced)*

- *Mozzarella Cheese (3 ½ oz)*

- *Green Olives (5, or to taste)*

- *Prosciutto (3 ½ oz, sliced)*

- *Olive Oil (3 tbsp)*

- *Salt (to taste)*

- *Pepper (to taste)*

How it's Made:

- Slice the tomato lengthwise, thinly.

- Slice the prosciutto.

- Assemble the sliced tomato pieces and the prosciutto onto a plate, adding in the green olives and mozzarella cheese. Drizzle with olive oil, and sprinkle with salt and pepper according to taste.

- Serve, and Enjoy!

Lunch

Asian Salad

This recipe makes 1 serving and requires about 20 minutes.

The serving size is 1 plate; it contains:

34 g Protein

7 g Carbs

98 g Fats

What's in It

For the Beef:

- *Ribeye steaks (⅓ lb)*

- *Ginger (½ tbsp, grated)*

- *Olive oil (½ tbsp)*

- *Chili Flakes (to taste)*

For the mayonnaise and sesame dressing:

- *Egg (1 yolk)*

- *Dijon mustard (½ tsp)*

- *Sesame oil (½ tbsp)*

- *Olive Oil (4 tbsp)*

- *Lime (1, juiced. Use ¼ tablespoon)*

- *Salt (to taste)*

- *Pepper (to taste)*

Alternative Dressing (if you would prefer not to make the dressing from scratch)

- *To your favorite brand of mayonnaise, squeeze in some lime juice and sesame oil, and mix until fully incorporated.*

For the Salad

- *Scallion (1, chopped)*

- *Red onion (¼)*

- *Cucumber (1 oz)*

- *Lettuce (1½ oz)*

- *Cherry tomatoes (1½ oz)*

- *Sesame seeds (a sprinkle)*

- *Cilantro (lightly chopped)*

How it's Made:

- First, make the mayonnaise and sesame dressing. Mix the egg yolk and the mustard in a bowl. Whisk together and pour in the olive oil as you continue to whisk. Stir in the spices, sesame seeds, and sesame oil. Set aside.

- Now for the beef. In a separate bowl, mix in the ginger, olive oil, and chili flakes. Pour the mixture into a plastic bag, and then add in the beef. Allow marinating for about 15 minutes.

- As the beef marinades, prepare the salad by chopping up the vegetables.

- Transfer the salad to a plate.

- In a medium frying pan, toast the sesame seeds for a couple of minutes on medium heat.

- Set the sesame seeds aside and pat the meat dry. Cook the meat on both sides on high heat, until it has cooked to your preference.

- Once cooked, remove the meat from the pan. Thinly slice, and place on top of the salad. Garnish with the toasted sesame seeds.

- Serve with the mayonnaise sesame dressing on the side.

Dinner

Ham Omelet with Herbs

This recipe makes 2 serving and requires about 15 minutes.

The serving size is 1 omelet; it contains:

51 g Protein

10.2 g Carbs

52.9 g Fats

What's in It

- *Eggs (4)*
- *Swiss Cheese (1 cup, shredded)*
- *Ham (4 oz, chopped)*
- *Scallions (2, chopped)*
- *Pepper (to taste)*
- *Salt (to taste)*
- *Dill (optional)*

How it's Made

- Grease a skillet with some cooking spray or butter. Beat the eggs in a separate bowl.

- Pour the eggs into the skillet. After about 5 minutes, or when the eggs have cooked, add the Swiss cheese and ham. Garnish with scallions and dill, if desired. Sprinkle with some salt and pepper.

- Serve, and enjoy!

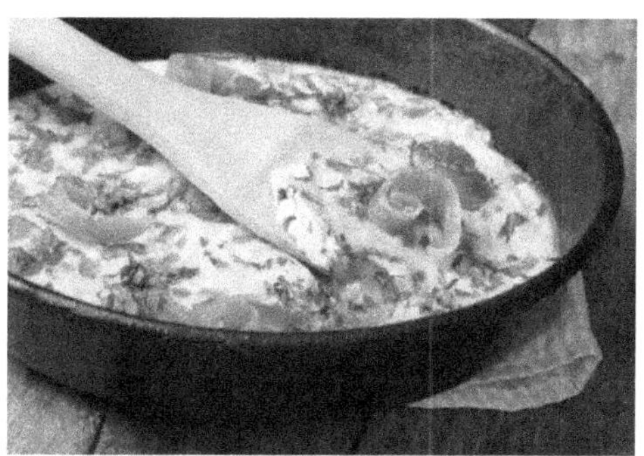

Day 13

Breakfast

Keto-Style Porridge

This recipe makes 1 serving and requires about 5 minutes.

The serving size is 1 bowl; it contains:

9 g Protein

4 g Carbs

49 g Fats

What's in It

- *Egg (1)*

- *Butter (1 oz) -- Alternative Coconut Oil*

- *Coconut Flour (1 oz)*

- *Coconut Cream (4 tbsp)*

- *Fresh Berries (to taste)*

-

How it's Made

- In a non-stick saucepan over low heat, add the egg, butter (or coconut oil), coconut flour, and cream. Stir until the porridge reaches the consistency that you wish.

- When the porridge is ready to your liking, transfer onto a separate plate. Top with some extra cream and some berries.

- Serve, and enjoy!

Lunch

Turkey Plate

This recipe makes 1 serving and requires about 5 minutes.

The serving size is 1 plate; it contains:

24 g Protein

9 g Carbs

75 g Fats

What's in It

- *Avocado (1)*

- *Deli Turkey (3 oz, sliced)*

- *Lettuce (1 oz)*

- *Olive Oil (to taste -- at least 2 tbsp)*

- *Cream Cheese (to taste -- at least 1 oz)*

- *Salt (to taste)*

- *Pepper (to taste)*

How it's Made

- Assemble the sliced turkey onto a plate.

- Slice the avocado and chop the lettuce. Place next to the turkey.

- Add a portion of cream cheese on the side.

- Sprinkle with salt and pepper.

- Drizzle over with olive oil, to taste.

- Serve, and enjoy!

Dinner

Simple Smoked Salmon with Spinach

This recipe makes 1 serving and requires about 5 minutes.

The serving size is 1 glass; it contains:

1058 g Protein

1 g Carbs

109 g Fats

What's in It

- *Baby Spinach (⅙ oz, or a handful)*

- *Smoked Salmon (6 oz)*

- *Mayonnaise (½ cup, or to taste)*

- *Olive Oil (to taste)*

- *Lemon, or lime-- according to taste. (cut into wedges)*

- *Salt (to taste)*

- *Pepper (to taste)*

How it's Made

- On a plate, assemble the smoked salmon, the baby spinach, and the mayonnaise.

- Cut the lemon (or lime) into wedges and add to the plate. Squeeze onto the salmon and spinach, according to taste. Sprinkle salt and pepper according to taste. Drizzle olive oil.

- Serve, and enjoy!

Day 14

Breakfast

Morning Smoothie

This recipe makes 2 servings and requires about 5 minutes.

The serving size is 1 glass; it contains:

3.68 g Protein

11.64 g Carbs

40.1 g Fats

What's in It

- *Avocado (½, frozen)*

- *Coconut Milk (1 cup)*

- *Almond Butter (1 tbsp)*

- *Cacao Powder (2 tsp)*

- *Coconut Oil (1 tbsp)*

- *Chia Seeds (1 tbsp, soaked in 3 tbsp of water for 10 minutes)*

- *Cinnamon (optional, for the top of the smoothie)*

- *Ice (optional)*

How it's Made

- In a high power blender like the Vitamix, add in the avocado, the coconut milk, almond butter, cacao powder, coconut oil, and soaked chia seeds. If you wish, add in some ice.

- Blend together until smooth.

- Pour into a glass, top with some extra cacao powder or cinnamon if desired.

- Serve, and enjoy!

Lunch

Simple Garden Salad (with or without a side of salmon)

What's in It

- *Romaine Lettuce (1 head)*

- *Grape tomatoes (9, sliced in half)*

- *Cucumber (1, chopped)*

- *Red Onion (1, thinly sliced)*

- *Olive Oil (to taste)*

- *Red Wine Vinegar (to taste)*

- *Salt (to taste)*

- *Pepper (to taste)*

How it's Made:

- Tear the romaine lettuce leaves into pieces and put into a salad bowl.

- Add the grape tomatoes, the cucumbers, and the onion.

- Add the olive oil and vinegar dressing according to taste and toss the salad together until it's all coated with the dressing.

- Sprinkle with salt and pepper.

- Serve, and Enjoy!

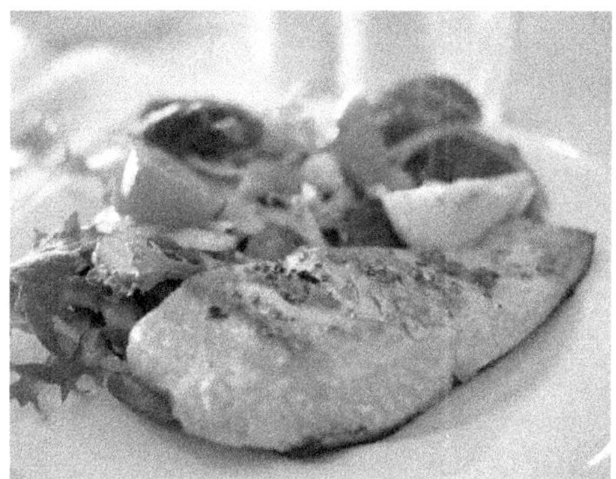

Dinner

Pizza and Side Salad

This recipe makes 1 serving and requires about 30 minutes.

The serving size is 1 pizza; it contains:

55 g Protein

8 g Carbs

90 g Fats

What's in It

For the Crust

- *Mozzarella Cheese (3 oz, shredded)*

- *Eggs (2)*

For the Toppings and Serving

- *Shredded Cheese (2 ½ oz)*

- *Tomato Paste (1 ½ tbsp)*

- *Olives (to taste)*

- *Pepperoni (¾ oz)*

- *Oregano (½ tsp)*

Side Salad

- *Leafy greens (romaine, a handful)*

- *Olive Oil (to taste)*

- *Lemon (½, juiced)*

- *Salt (to taste)*

- *Pepper (to taste)*

How it's Made

- Preheat the oven to 400 degrees Fahrenheit.

- Make the crust by cracking the eggs into a bowl and mixing in the cheddar cheese.

- Line a baking sheet with parchment paper. Spread the egg and cheese mixture onto it. Form the mix into a round circular shape, or a rectangular shape according to your choice.

- Bake the pizza crust in the oven for about 15 minutes, or until it turns golden.

- When the crust is ready, take it out of the oven and let it cool.

- Increase the oven's temperature to 450 degrees Fahrenheit.

- As the oven's temperature increases, spread the tomato paste onto the pizza crust, and add on the toppings.

- Place back into the oven, and bake for another 15-20 minutes, until the pizza turns a golden brown.

- Let the pizza cool, and transfer to another plate.

- Prepare the fresh romaine salad on the side by tossing the leaves in some fresh lemon juice and olive oil. Sprinkle with salt and pepper on the top.

- Serve and enjoy!

Conclusion

Thanks for making it through to the end of *Keto for Beginners: Essentials to Get Started with the Ketogenic Diet and Reset Your Metabolism in 14 Days*, let's hope it was informative and able to provide you with all of the tools you need to achieve your goals whatever they may be.

The next step is to continue exploring the ketogenic diet, so you can continue to discover the numerous health benefits, experiment with a variety of nutritious and fun recipes, and enjoy the life-long benefits of a healthy weight and a vibrant body.

Finally, if you found this book useful in any way, a review on Amazon is always appreciated!